Cor

The Incredible Power of the Power Nap: Your Guide to a 'Quickie'

Deep Sleep:

32 Proven Tips for Deeper, Longer, More Rejuvenating Sleep

By C.K. Murray

Similar works by C.K. Murray:

Mindfulness Explained: The Mindful Solution to Stress, Depression, and Chronic Unhappiness

Vitamin D Explained: The Incredible, Healing Powers of Sunlight

The Confidence Cure: Your Definitive Guide to Overcoming Low Self-Esteem, Learning Self-Love and Living Happily

The Stress Fallacy: Why Everything You Know Is WRONG

High Blood Pressure Explained: Natural, Effective, Drug-Free Treatment for the "Silent Killer"

ADHD Explained: Natural, Effective, Drug-Free Treatment For Your Child

You close your eyes, your breathing slows. Somewhere, the thoughts quiet and the voices soften. Visions from earlier begin to fade. Your pulse is low; your muscles loose. You, my friend, are falling to sleep.

But sometimes, it isn't *nearly* so easy.

On planet Earth, all living organisms must sleep. While patterns and reasons for sleep may vary from organism to organism, species to species, the act itself is a constant. Universally, sleep is crucial. It is believed to rejuvenate our bodies and minds, preparing us for the demands of every new day. Some of us get a lot, some very little. Although we all do it and we all *need* to do it, few of us understand it. What does it mean, when we slip into that dark, mysterious world? What happens once that curtain is pulled and we're no longer consciously in control?

Or are we?

When it comes to sleep, understanding the nature of the function is almost as tough as understanding the strange dreams that come within it. The questions are always coming too. What is sleep, really? Why do we sometimes wake up in the middle? Why is it deeper one night and shallow the next? And how much do we really need of it? Is there a set number? Can we program our bodies and minds to get enough?

Why can some people get it with ease, while others can struggle their entire lives just to catch a wink?

These are just some of the most basic questions that sleep experts are tackling. With every new study—every new thought—the light grows. And with great hope, it bestows in the dark a little piece of the puzzle.

When it comes to everyday things, the effects of sleep are most obvious when we're *not* getting it. Getting proper rest is essential because it maintains normal cognitive functioning in speech, memory, and fluid thinking. Basically, it plays a significant role in normal brain development. When we aren't sleeping adequately, we experience a host of physical and mental issues. With continued lack of good sleep, the part of the brain that controls language, memory, planning and sense of time begins to power down.

Studies show that 17 hours of sustained wakefulness leads to diminished cognitive and physical performance equivalent to a blood alcohol level of 0.05%. In other words, if you stay up for 17 hours, all other factors controlled, you'll feel like you've had two glasses of wine. More than this, continued and consistent lack of quality sleep can lead to more serious problems like diabetes, depression, cardiovascular disease, and obesity. The risk of chronic illness skyrockets as a result of sleep deprivation.

And this should be no surprise. Seeing as the human being spends nearly a third of its life asleep, there is no denying the importance of rest on good health and wellbeing. But again, what are the exact reasons for this function? Becoming unconscious during sleep is something we seem to just accept... but why? What is actually going *on* in there?

What Happens When We Sleep?

Upon waking, we usually won't remember much about those hours that passed. Sometimes we'll come to, feeling as if it was no more than a wink. Other times, we'll feel as if we're returning from a distant world. For the most part, though, people don't really think about what happened. We lie down, at some point we drift off, and then we wake up. Maybe we can account for dreams, or times during the night where we tossed and turned, but usually, it's more or less a blur.

Even so, if we want to understand how to improve the quality and quantity of our sleep, we need to understand what makes sleep, *sleep*. The defining traits of sleep are:

- A period of reduced activity

- In humans, posture such as lying down with the eyes closed

- A diminished responsiveness to external stimuli

- A state relatively easy to reverse, opposed to hibernation or coma

Sleep is basically a period where the body and mind are less concerned with external processes, and more concerned with *internal* processes. Although we are not consciously aware of these processes while sleeping, they are certainly notable. During the hours of necessary rest, our bodies and brains are undergoing very real, very intriguing physical changes.

These include:

Brain Activity – Physicians believed for the longest time that the brain became inactive during sleep. However, in the past 6 decades this myth has been dispelled. While there *is* a progressive decrease in the "firing" rate of many neurons in the brain as sleep progresses, there is certainly something still going on 'up there.' In fact, studies show that the activity during sleep is much more choreographed, shall we say, than during wakefulness.

During REM sleep, the stage of sleep linked to dreaming, there is a dramatic increase in brain activity. This is because REM sleep is a period of rest where there is high cortical activity, and almost no consciousness of the environment. The eyes are rapidly moving during this period and the skeletal muscles are paralyzed, preventing you from acting out your dreams. In some cases, the brain is actually more active during REM sleep than it would be during our most mentally stimulating wakeful moment. So if you think your dreams are "crazy," there's a good reason why... Your brain is on rapid fire!

Interestingly, this level of activity seems specific to humans. Our entire brains are involved in the sleeping process, but in other animals, a certain degree of consciousness remains, meaning that only a portion of their brains are dedicated to sleep. Perhaps if we had to constantly be on the look-out for predators, our brains would work the same way. Fortunately, that is not the case.

Physiological Changes – There are countless biological processes occurring both in sleep and wakefulness. During sleep, our processes are typically reduced, including temperature and blood pressure. When we are in REM sleep, the state associated with dreaming, our processes are likely to be highly varied. Temperature, oxygen circulation, carbon dioxide, and blood glucose are all acting on various levels. However, when we are in non-REM sleep, the non-dream state, our levels are extremely regularized. During this phase, we tend to—as they say—sleep soundly. There is no consciousness of the environment, little cortical activity, and virtually no internal thoughts.

Non-REM or NREM sleep consists of three stages: N1 (light sleep), N2, and N3 (that deep sleep where a bomb going off couldn't wake you). Sleep proceeds in cycles of REM and NREM, with four or five per night. The order is typically N1 → N2 → N3 → N2 → REM. We all go through more N3 deep sleep earlier in the night, and the amount of REM sleep increases in two cycles immediately prior to natural awakening.

Cardiovascular Changes – Your heart is pretty wild, isn't it? Well during sleep, this magnificent pump goes through two phases. In non-REM sleep, blood pressure and pulse go down. Your body is at rest and your heart is recovering from the day. During REM sleep, though, your blood pressure and heart rate are sometimes jacked. Interestingly, males will often get erections and females, clitoral swelling, both a believed result of nervous system changes and responses to dreams.

Respiratory Levels – Speaking of physiological changes, a lot of what happens in our body during sleep has to do with our breathing. When awake, breathing is usually quite irregular. Think about it. You are being physically active, or not—you are stressed, you are relaxed; your speech, emotions, posture, and activity levels all affect your breathing. But when we are progressing through non-REM sleep, our respiratory efforts decrease and stabilize. Of course, when we enter the dream stage of REM sleep, those wild and crazy imaginings jack our breathing back up.

Upswing in Physiological *Activity* – This one might be a little confusing. After all, even if our brains are active during dream phase, aren't we lying still during sleep? How could our physiological activity go *up*? Well, it's pretty simple. Most physiological activities are decreased—you're right. But some, such as the release of growth hormone, go up. This happens because the body and mind are likely trying to repair and restore certain functions. Activities linked to digestion, cell repair, and growth typically reach their peak during sleep, suggesting that cell repair, regrowth, and rejuvenation may be central features of sleeping. Not to mention, we're still burning calories while asleep, and for some of us—all that tossing, turning, and limb movement is akin to a workout!

Now that you're aware of some of the important changes that occur during sleep, you are probably aware of two important truths: (1) the brain and body are far from inactive during sleep, and (2) these activity levels are central to the purpose of sleep. But now that creates more questions. Such as, why are these changes actually occurring? What do they mean and why? Is there a sole primary function of sleep, or does sleep serve many?

Although there is no surefire consensus regarding the purpose of sleep, many have come to several presiding theories. By understanding these theories, we are all better prepared for higher quality sleep, and a healthier, happier life.

Why Do We Sleep? Understanding the Multiple Theories of a Good Night's Sleep

There are a lot of theories out there concerning the exact purpose of sleep. Although it is easy for some of them to overlap, there are definitely distinctions among them all. For the longest time, sleep experts and scientists have argued over the credibility of various points, drawing comparisons to other creatures and their sleeping patterns. While this is an important part of scientific discovery, perhaps it is best to let humans be humans. After all, what other creatures on this planet can dream up the incredible worlds that we can?

For now, here are the four dominant sleep theories, and their explanations:

Inactivity Theory or "Adaptive" Theory

This is one of the oldest theories of sleep, also called the evolutionary theory. It essentially suggests that inactivity during the night is an adaptation that works as a survival mechanism by keeping organisms away from harm. Because organisms would normally be harmed during this period, sleep ensures that they go unseen. Instead of moving about during the night and making a mistake or being caught off guard by a predator, sleeping animals are very still and quiet.

Through natural selection, this behavioral strategy is believed to evolve to what we now recognize as sleep. The Inactivity Theory is supported by studies of animals with many predators and those with few, such as bears and lions. In the case of those with few, sleep occurs for long periods, oftentimes during the day. For animals with numerous predators, sleep only lasts for the most vulnerable periods of the night. Of course, this theory can be quickly argued if we only consider one thing: animals are better prepared for protecting themselves if they are conscious. Being unconscious may be good for not making a lot of noise or motion, but once that unconscious animal is discovered by a predator—its safety is compromised.

Restorative Theory

This one is interesting if not for the simple fact that it supposes that good rest really does make every day a 'new' day. This theory implies that sleep restores what we lose every day in all our pressing thoughts, behaviors, and emotions. Recently, empirical evidence from human and animal studies has shown that animals completely deprived of sleep lose *all* immune function and die in mere weeks. These findings are further supported by research that shows the major restorative functions in the sleeping body including muscle growth, tissue repair, protein synthesis, and growth hormone.

When it comes to other restorative properties of sleep, the brain is central.

When awake, accumulation of neurons in the brain produces adenosine, a cellular by-product. With enough adenosine, we begin to perceive of feelings of tiredness and weakness. Thus it is no surprise that caffeine has been shown to block the actions of this by-product in the brain. As long as we are awake, adenosine accumulates and remains high. When sleeping, however, the body clears it from the system and we feel much more alert. Adenosine may very well be one of the chemical reasons behind the sleep drive. It is believed that neurotoxins and waste products that accumulate in the central nervous system during the day are flushed out through sleep. This may also help shed light on the processes that lead to, and prevent, cognitive degenerative conditions like Alzheimer's.

Brain Plasticity

This theory is the most recent and compelling as far as science is concerned. According to this one, sleep is correlated with very real changes in the structure and organization of the human brain. Brain plasticity refers to the brain's ability to readily adapt and self-modify, in accordance with various other internal and external demands. Although not entirely comprehensible, its connection to sleep has several critical implications. It is becoming clear, for example, that sleep plays a most important role in brain development in both infants and young kids. Infants spend roughly 13 to 14 hours a day sleeping, with half that time in the dreamscapes of REM sleep. The link between sleep and brain plasticity is also revealing itself in adults, as studies show that chronic sleep deprivation restructures the brain. Ultimately, this impacts a person's ability to learn and perform a massive range of tasks.

Now that you have a more nuanced understanding of the various theories of sleep, it's time to delve deeper. Let's take these theories and apply them to that important thing that makes the human brain so amazing. That's right—*learning*.

When it comes to making sense of sleep and dreams, and the mind and body's incredible powers, we'd be remiss if we didn't consider learning. The human brain is remarkably adaptive, rewiring its neurons, changing its chemical levels, and restructuring its assets when the time calls.

If you're hoping to use sleep to improve your memory, boost your cognitive performance, and enhance your waking mind—now's the time!

Sleep and Learning: How Sleep Rebuilds the Brain

We've all been there. We're sitting at work, sitting in class, somewhere, doing some*thing*, and all we can do is think about how tired we are. Maybe we think, *gosh I need a coffee*. Or maybe we opt for some energy drink like Redbull or Rockstar. Or maybe, simply, we find a nice place to curl up and catch some shuteye. The bottom line is: we're fatigued. And the reason we're fatigued is because we need rest, we need sleep. When humans go without sleep too long, the brain and body suffer. The brain specifically loses its ability to focus, and thus, its ability to learn. And the effects go on… without sleep, we can no longer take advantage of that nice time to unwind, and our brains—fighting for some 'clean-up' time—can no longer perform one of their most vital functions: memory consolidation.

Learning and memory include the following critical terms:

Acquisition – the introduction of new information

Consolidation -- the processes that make a memory stable

Recall – the ability to access information after storage, whether conscious or unconscious

All three steps must occur for memory and learning to take place. Although acquisition and recall happen only when we are awake, memory consolidation happens during sleep. Think about it. According to the Brain Plasticity theory, our brains are restructuring and rewiring during sleep, in part due to what happened during the day. When this happens, certain neural networks create new memories. In rough terms, think of learning as exercise. When you exercise and work out your muscles, your muscles temporarily break down. They are stimulated, challenged, and weakened. However, once you rest, those specific muscles are strengthened. Same thing applies to your neurons. You flex your neurons, you stimulate them, they are challenged and stretched and pulled and jerked—and then, when your mind is given the time it needs—those neurons come back stronger.

In strengthening or weakening neural pathways, there are several factors. Depending upon the different stages of sleep, changes in sleep duration, and changes in the amount of sleep, the ability to learn different tasks is affected. More specifically, memory of learned material is correlated directly with many sleep stages.

One type of memory correlated frequently with sleep stages is *declarative memory*. This type of memory is the knowledge of fact-based information, or "what" we know. Examples include remembering what you ate for breakfast, the name of a capital city, or your home address. Relating to sleep stages, several studies have shown that language courses often trigger our declarative memories. In fact, students of intensive language courses typically spend more time in REM sleep, meaning that their brains are at an accelerated level of cortical activity.

Research asserts that REM sleep is usually most applicable when learned information has a strong emotional component and is complex. Simple, emotionally flat information is not linked to REM sleep. Other features of sleep have also been linked to declarative memory consolidation. Researchers believe that slow-wave sleep (SWS), or deep, restorative sleep, forms a significant role in this type of memory by processing and consolidating fresh info.

These stages of sleep have also been associated with other types of memory. For instance, procedural memory, which reminds us how to do something, is also consolidated through REM sleep. When you get in your car and drive, or prepare your morning cup of coffee, procedural memory is critical. Other types, such as visual learning, are also linked to the amount and onset of slow-wave sleep and REM sleep. Motor learning, by contrast, depends on the amount of lighter stages of sleep such as N1. In general, the various types of memory depend largely on the amount of sleep, the stage of sleep, and the time of that sleep. Although the connections are still complicated, and the research still underdeveloped, we *are* getting closer.

Sleep Deprivation and Performance

The different stages of sleep are only good for memory if they are adequate in length and depth. When we are sleep deprived, our focus, attention, and vigilance deplete, and receiving new information becomes very hard. Lacking adequate sleep and rest, our strained neurons can no longer function, can no longer coordinate information properly, and ultimately lose their ability to access learned information. This also affects our interpretation of events. We can't recall with clarity, we can't make sound decisions, we can't accurately assess problems, we can't plan, we can't react, and we generally can't employ good judgment. Basically, sleep deprivation affects all aspects of our being.

If being chronically tired to the point of fatigue or exhaustion sounds bad, just think about your emotional wellbeing. Neurons, muscles, and organ systems aside, lack of sleep will dramatically impact your mood. Changes in mood, whether subtle or drastic, can leave us feeling incapable of learning. We will not acquire new information as seamlessly, and will not remember that information as easily. Mood swings can become common, and a general groggy, depressive affect is not unheard of. It is quite clear that a good night's rest has a significant impact on learning and memory.

But that's not all…

Your Life Depends On It! Major Health Problems Caused by Sleep Deprivation AND Oversleeping

Don't let the outliers in your life fool you. Sure, there's always going to be somebody who claims they can function fine on minimal sleep—and maybe they can. Even so, sleep is a necessary component of life. The average person requires 7-9 hours a night, and though some may seem sprightly off a measly 4, others might need 10 or even 11 to feel right. Sleep needs vary from person to person, but what doesn't vary is the importance of sleep. Even if you have 'adapted' to sleeping very little, that doesn't mean your body and mind are doing fine.

There is a wealth of research showing the connection between sleep habits and the risk of developing diseases. Firstly, *sleep deprivation studies* take participants and study acute reactions to lack of sleep over short periods. The early effects are then correlated with the possible onset of more long-term diseases. In most cases, these participants show higher blood pressure, reduced control of blood glucose, and worsened inflammation. These effects are associated with stress and can become unmanageable over time.

Secondly, *epidemiological studies* take questionnaires distributed to large populations and assess the responses. Those lacking in sleep typically report a significantly higher incidence of hypertension, diabetes, and obesity. These studies, of course, do no show causation, but do display a correlation.

Finally, *longitudinal studies* track sleep habits and disease issues in individuals over time. By starting with people who are initially disease-free, these studies reveal how the time of disease onset, changes in severity, and changes in sleep patterns interact in specific individuals. By understanding population patterns, individual cases, and self-reported interactions, sleep specialists are gaining a greater understanding of the many health problems associated with inadequate sleep.

Let's familiarize ourselves with these health problems:

Diabetes

Inadequate sleep also leads to type 2 diabetes. This happens because the body is influenced by the way it processes glucose, which is the high-energy carbohydrate that cells need. Studies have shown that even in healthy subjects, when sleep is cut back from 8 to 4 hours per night, participants processed glucose more slowly than they did when they were allowed to sleep longer. Many epidemiological studies have shown that adults who sleep less than five hours a night are at a much greater risk of getting diabetes. Obstructive sleep apnea has also been linked to diabetes.

Obesity

If you don't like being overweight, you better start getting some sleep.

More than a few studies have linked insufficient sleep with weight gain.

In fact, people who habitually sleep less under six hours per night are significant inclined to have higher than average body mass indexes (BMI). Moreover, those who sleep eight hours show the lowest BMI. Lack of sleep is now considered as responsible for obesity as poor diet and sedentary lifestyle.

Sleep helps to control weight a number of ways. When we're out, our bodies secrete hormones that control appetite, metabolism, and glucose levels. Obtaining too little sleep upsets the balance of these and other hormones. If you are getting inadequate sleep, your body produces more of the stress hormone, cortisol, which leads to general poor health when chronically induced. In excessive amounts, cortisol can even break down skin collagen, the protein that keeps our flesh elastic and looking nice.

Furthermore, poor sleep is also linked to the production of insulin, which exacerbates weight gain and diabetes. If that isn't bad enough, you've got more to worry about. Inadequate sleep causes your brain to produce less leptin. When there is less leptin in your body, your brain does not recognize the feeling of 'fullness' as it should. Not to mention, ghrelin is produced in excess, causing an increase in appetite. This means that poor sleep may cause us to want more food, even when we've already met our calorie needs. This is a multi-layered problem. In the end, we end up gaining weight more because we're more stressed, our mind can't determine if we've had enough, our appetite is inflated, and our bodies are too tired to do any exercising that would burn off the fat. Throw on the fact that sleep deprivation reduces human growth hormone—important for muscle growth—and you've got a recipe for weight gain.

Heart Disease and Hypertension

Hypertension is believed to afflict 1 in 3 Americans. In cultures that pride salty diets, the rates may be significantly higher. And when it comes to hypertension, or high blood pressure, heart disease is not far off.

Studies show that even minor periods of inadequate sleep can jack up the blood pressure.

A single night of inadequate sleep in people with hypertension has been shown to cause elevated blood pressure throughout the entire next day. Some studies have found that sleeping too little (less than six hours) or excessively (more than nine hours) significantly increases the risk of coronary heart disease in women. In short, sleep is crucial when it comes to cardiovascular health.

Mounting evidence also shows that obstructive sleep apnea and heart disease are highly linked. Those suffering from sleep apnea will typically awake multiple times during the night. This happens because their airways close when they fall asleep. Apnea sufferers also experience acute spikes in blood pressure every time they wake up. Over time, these episodes lead to hypertension, which puts them at major risk for cardiovascular disease. In short, inadequate sleep increases the risk of:

- Heart disease

- Heart attack

- Heart failure

- Irregular heartbeat

- High blood pressure

- Stroke

- Diabetes

Sounds like fun doesn't it?

Mood Disorders

This one is a no-brainer. Without question, you've met somebody who was cranky or irritable or prone to mood swings due to crummy sleep. Chances are, you've been this person—we all have. But what if chronic insufficient sleep actually leads to more than just moodiness, but actual mood disorders?

Well, studies show that it does. Chronic sleep issues are correlated with depression, anxiety, and mental distress, maladies that are often treated through cognitive behavioral therapy and medication. Studies have shown that people who sleep four and a half hours each night report feeling greater levels of stress, sadness, anger, and mental exhaustion. Other studies have linked scant sleep with diminished levels of optimism and sociability. Inadequate sleep has even been associated with reduced sex drive. Fortunately, returning to a normal sleep schedule fixes all these problems.

Alcohol Abuse

Many people may have a few drinks to 'unwind.' Unfortunately, studies show that alcohol is actually bad for sleep in the long-term. Consuming alcohol causes sleep disturbances and poor sleeping patterns, especially in habitual drinkers. When it comes to alcohol, it goes both ways. Alcohol use is more prevalent among those who sleep poorly and those who drink alcohol typically sleep poorly. Although the mild sedative effects of alcohol may help people with insomnia, the effects are only temporary. After alcohol is processed by the body, it begins to stimulate the brain in order to trigger arousal. This is why drinkers usually get up in the middle of the night, toss and turn, or wake up before they are well rested.

Accident Prevalence

This one is obvious, and we all try to deal with it as best we can. For most people, a morning cup of coffee is the answer. Even so, sleep deprivation has been linked with many major accidents, including the nuclear accident at Three Mile Island, the Exxon Valdez oil spill, and several other headline-grabbing disasters.

On the everyday road, drowsiness causes slow reaction time—similar to driving while intoxicated. The National Highway Traffic Safety Administration approximates sleep deprivation as a cause in 100,000 automobile every year in the United States. Off the road and on the job, lack of sleep is equally problematic. Workers who complain of excessive sleepiness often have significantly more work-related accidents, and typically miss more work due to sick days.

Immune System Problems

When you're sick, you're usually tired. This is because the immune system produces sleep-inducing chemicals that also help fight infection. In relation to the various theories of sleep, immune functions shut down the body in order to trigger reparation and rejuvenation. Sick animals at sleep are more able to maintain normal functioning after sleeping than those who do not get adequate sleep. When we don't get enough sleep, our immune system is unlikely able to work as effectively.

Life Expectancy

After covering the various health issues linked to inadequate sleep, it is not surprising that poor sleep can lead to a reduced life expectancy. Data from large cross-sectional epidemiological studies shows that five hours or less per night increases mortality risk from all known causes by about 15 percent. Even so, it's important to remember that correlation does not imply causation. Poor sleep may bring on disease, but sometimes people with disease then experience poor sleep. Due to the lack of awareness of sleep issues, and the acceptance of sleep deprivation as a part of our frenzied modern worlds, it is no wonder that truly understanding sleep is a problem harder than most.

And when it comes to understanding this problem that is tougher than most, we have a lot of *sub-problems* to sift through. That's right, sleep disorders…

Basically, chronic inadequate sleep has serious effects on your life, some that may come on suddenly, some that may slowly build over time. Serious medical conditions like diabetes, high blood pressure, heart disease, and a shortened life expectancy all come from sleep issues. Moreover, sleeping in excess has *also* been shown to lead to many physical and mental health issues.

So don't risk it! Take the time to recover; *make* time to sleep.

Sleep Disorder

Every night, some 30 to 40 million Americans have difficulty getting to sleep, remaining asleep, or waking up earlier than they would like. It has been estimated that some 50 to 70 million Americans suffer from some type of sleep disorder, but these estimates may be low. This is due, of course, to the lack of reporting by many patients to their doctors. As a result, the widespread lack of awareness for sleep problems has costly and ugly repercussions for society. Loss of productivity and medical bills are just part of it.

The worst part, the most *intimate* part, is the cost to the individual. Studies show that individuals with sleep disorders are more prone to clinical depression, poor concentration, and accidents. The emotional, physical, and even spiritual toll that sleep disorders take on the human creature is incredible.

For people with sleep disorders, the mind and body are out-of-whack. The internal body clock is not cued into certain external factors such as light and dark. Normally people undergo "circadian rhythms," but in those with sleep disorders these rhythms are disrupted. Instead of producing melatonin when it's dark to wind down the mind and body, disordered individuals may struggle with chemical imbalance. They may also struggle with cortisol production in the morning to wake them up. And the list goes on.

Let's review, briefly, the troubling and tiring disorders of modern day sleep… and the ways to treat them:

Chronic Insomnia

Insomnia typically comes as a result of poor sleep habits. People who consume too much alcohol or caffeine near bedtime, or who expose themselves to strong electronic stimuli prior to bedtime, are likely to struggle with falling asleep. Antidepressants, allergy and cold products, and steroids also bring on insomnia. Chronic insomnia can also be a symptom of clinical psychiatric conditions such as anxiety disorders and major depression.

When there is no clear environmental, psychiatric, or medical cause attributed to insomnia, that insomnia is called "primary insomnia." In these cases, deviations in brain signaling and chemical processing may account for the sleeping issues.

In order to treat insomnia, a resolution of health issues or external factors usually suffices. If the issues are deeper than this, or more complicated, other treatment options exist:

Behavioral techniques

- Sleep hygiene, which includes regularizing one's bedtime and wake-up time, creating an environment conducive to sleep, and avoiding substances and behaviors (like extended naps) that can disrupt sleep

- Cognitive behavioral therapy (CBT) which addresses fears and insecurities of not falling asleep. CBT changes the attitudes one has toward sleep by impacting the relevant emotions and behaviors that affect, and are affected by, those attitudes

- Meditation and biofeedback to induce relaxation. Biofeedback teaches patients how to focus on their natural bodily rhythms (pulse, breathing, tension, etc.)

Pharmaceutical Options

- Hypnotics are the drugs most commonly prescribed for sleep issues. They are effective and can be used with antidepressants that also promote sleep

- Over the counter drugs are also effective at times, including antihistamines, which cause drowsiness. Herbal sleep remedies may also be effective, but the evidence is inconclusive

Some of these may be successful in individual cases. Sleep aids often contain an antihistamine, which causes sleepiness but also can cause daytime drowsiness. Of the many herbal sleep remedies promoted as sleep aids, none have been conclusively found to be effective.

Excessive Daytime Sleepiness (EDS)

Yes, this is actually considered a serious problem when it becomes an everyday thing. Statistics show that 60% of adult drivers have driven a vehicle drowsy; most alarming, however, is that more than a third have actually fallen asleep at the wheel.

Having trouble staying awake is one thing, but suddenly falling to sleep is not normal—and is the mark of EDS. Excessive Daytime Sleepiness is present in most sleep disorders, such as obstructive sleep apnea, narcolepsy, and limb movement disorders.

Obstructive Sleep Apnea (OSA)

Imagine the most disruptive snoring you can envision. In this case, the individual's airway becomes partially or completely blocked throughout the night, causing many awakenings. Because sleep causes the muscles in the throat to relax, for some people, this relaxation leads to blockage. In some people, this relaxation causes tissue at the back of the throat to block the airway. In extreme forms of OSA, this blockage can occur hundreds of times during the night. It can interrupt breathing for half a minute every time.

Despite all of these awakenings, most people with OSA don't remember the events. Only daytime fatigue and reports from partners make OSA known to the individual. For this reason, OSA should not be taken lightly. It can lead to hypertension, heart disease, and mood and memory issues.

Treatment

- Weight loss is likely the best treatment for OSA. Shedding pounds may lessen or even eliminate the disorder. Obesity causes OSA because excessive weight typically increases the amount of tissue in the throat, making airway obstruction likelier. Inherited traits such as small jaw size or big overbite, and excessive use of alcohol before sleep can contribute to OSA.

- Continuous positive airway pressure (CPAP) is also an effective treatment option for people with moderate to severe OPA. During sleep, a handy little device keeps the airway open by sending a consistent, low-pressure airstream through the nose and into the airway.

- Position therapy is a basic, non-invasive option. Although it is not that effective, it is easy to implement. Typically position therapy features a change of position (duh!). Some people can sleep on their side and reduce or eliminate the symptoms. Others cannot. Still, it's worth a shot.

- Dental devices are a more invasive option that reposition the lower jaw in a way that opens the airway consistently. This can work well for those with moderate to severe cases.

- The most drastic measures are surgical procedures. They typically widen the airway and prevent constriction.

- As yet, no medications have been shown to be effective in treating OSA.

Narcolepsy

This disorder is the one often depicted in comedy flicks. It is best known as a desperate need to fall asleep at all different locations all throughout the daytime. However, these "sleep attacks" are not as typical as one would think. Usually narcolepsy is about excessive daytime sleepiness. It affects roughly one in two thousand people, and is a central nervous system disorder in which the brain does not adequately regulate cycles of sleep and wakefulness. In the end, sleep is disturbed, and sufferers are incapable of staying awake for too long.

Narcolepsy also leads to cataplexy. Basically, cataplexy is the onset of sudden muscle weakness and, sometimes, manifests as a reversible paralysis in the appendages or face. It can sometimes cause a person to fall down, appear sleepy, and/or remain temporarily paralyzed while conscious. Narcolepsy also sometimes leads to hypnagogic hallucinations, which are dream-like experiences that happen when drifting into sleep. Sleep paralysis also occurs when waking up and falling asleep. In these cases, the inability to talk or move is briefly gone.

Treatment

Daytime sleeping assessments and nighttime studies are required to diagnose narcolepsy. Although there is no known cure, narcolepsy is typically treated with stimulants and antidepressants that prevent paralytic and hallucinatory symptoms. Scheduling convenient daytime naps may also help to overcome "sleep attacks."

Periodic Limb Movements of Sleep (PLMS)

This is a weird one, along the lines of "restless leg syndrome." Basically, it's a condition affecting over one-third of adults over 60. It causes involuntary kicking and jerking of the legs and arms, usually done more than a hundred times throughout the night. People with PLMS are usually unaware of their nighttime awakenings unless notified by a partner. When the symptoms make sleep so crappy that they contribute to daytime sleepiness, the condition is upgraded to disorder status. The name for this is **Periodic Limb Movement Disorder (PLMD)**.

Treatment

Because PLMD features a lot of motor issues, it is typically treated with medications applied to Parkinson's disease. Sleeping pills may also be used.

Parasomnias

These disorders are scary and odd, ranging from a pure fear of falling asleep, to horrific, baffling behaviors that are not remembered. People who experience parasomnias oftentimes don't even want to go to sleep. Many times, this only makes the conditions worse.

- Sleepwalking—You've heard of this one. People get up and walk around the house. Maybe they simply move about the hallway, or maybe they actually go to the closet and get redressed. Truth be told, sleepwalking actually takes place during deep non-REM sleep, so it is *not* an acting-out of dreams. Sleepwalkers like to perform routines, and are typically children. Only 1 percent of adults sleepwalk, and when they do, it is typically caused by anxiety, stress, or alcohol binges.

- Sleep-eating disorders—These also occur during deep sleep and signal partial awakenings. Individuals with these disorders will go downstairs and fix themselves sandwiches. They won't remember or know what they're doing.

- Night terrors—These are the most harrowing and severe of the parasomnias. They affect children, usually, and will cause a sudden bout of screams. Although these individuals may appear to have suffered tremendous fear or panic, they typically don't remember the episodes the next morning. However, when they are told about their odd sleep behaviors, sufferers will *then* begin to develop feelings of fear and insecurity.

Treatment

Self-hypnosis and/or sleep medications and antidepressants that prevent partial awakenings should be prescribed in certain cases. These cases typically include situations in which the sufferer is at risk of hurting him or herself and/or others. Night terrors that are frequent and impair daily functioning should be treated with more sleep medications, antidepressants, or relaxation techniques.

When it comes to sleepwalkers, sleep specialists will suggest ensuring that the environment is safe for everybody. This may be hard to do, and family members or friends should consult with experts and physicians to determine the suitable course of action for their particular case.

When it comes to sleep issues and disorders, there are certain things to consider. The rhythm and timing of the internal clock undergoes many changes with age. Teens fall asleep later than younger children and adults. Humans need more sleep early in life, during crucial development. This is why newborns may sleep more than 16 hours a day, and why preschoolers require naps. In some cases, individuals may outgrow sleep problems. In other cases, behavioral and cognitive interventions are necessary. In extreme cases, drug regimens may be the most effective.

But what about people in general? What about the man who can't fall asleep because he has a big meeting the next day, and he's stressed about his career, and he's got a house and mortgage, and bills are piling up, the kids are getting older, and his wife is pregnant with another child?

Or what about the woman who can't stop thinking about her less-than-perfect life? The one who can't unwind, who feels like *forever* since she's actually enjoyed quality sleep? What about the adult who is getting by on caffeine fumes entirely?

Sound familiar?

32 Proven Tips for Deeper, Longer, More Rejuvenating Sleep

So let's say you toss and turn and struggle with getting quality sleep. Let's also say that you have every *intention* of getting quality sleep, but 'something' always comes up. Maybe it's your fault, or perhaps life just throws you a curveball out of the blue. Whatever the cause, lacking quality sleep on a regular basis is a tremendous pain in the ass. So let's alleviate the pain and get on the right track.

Here are 32 proven tips for catching those wonderful Zs you've been missing:

Turn your bedroom into a "*sleep room*"

Okay, that sounded a little hokey, but the main point is this: your mind and body need the right environment to induce sleep. Especially if you, like many people, are stressed and anxious. A quiet, dark, and cool environment is ideal. According to the Division of Sleep Medicine at Harvard Medical School, the perfect temperature is between 60 and 75°F. Our bodies go through natural pattern of highs and lows, dipping to their minimum temperature at roughly 5am—so be sure your room temperature is neither too hot or too cold. Using blankets can also help with this problem.

Because light is a powerful cue that tells the brain to wake up, you need to eliminate your exposure to that as well. Make sure to have a mattress and pillows that are right for you. Don't be afraid of spending too much time choosing a mattress for firmness or softness—same with the pillow. Also, remember that most mattresses wear out over a decade. Be sure to limit your bedroom activities to sleep and sex only. Keep electronics and work-related activities out of the bedroom.

This is called conditioning, and it works!

Bed Size

If your partner is taking too much of the bed, he or she is also taking too much of your sleep quality away. In fact, the Sleep Council warns that being disturbed by a partner is one of the most common reasons for poor sleep.

A big enough bed allows you to lie side by side with your arms behind your head and elbows out, without touching your partner. A standard double bed is 4ft 6in (135cm) wide, allowing each sleeper just over 2 ft of space in which to sleep. This is less than the width of a baby's cot, and is not adequate. Many studies reveal that couples sleep better in bigger beds. A king-sized bed might just be a worthy investment.

Go Wool

The typical person loses a liter of water through sweat every night. Unfortunately, sweat cannot be absorbed through down or synthetic types of bedding. Over time, that moisture buildup on the skin may wake you up or diminish sleep quality. To combat this, use Duvets and pillows with wool filling that can draw sweat away from the body and trap it inside the fibers. This regulates the body temperature, making for longer, deeper, more satisfying sleep.

Chamomile Tea

Let's be honest, you've got a lot on your mind. If life is hurrying by and your mind is reeling, maybe it's time to decompress. One of the best ways to do so, studies show, is through the simple enjoyment of a cup of tea. In fact, chamomile herbal drink has been shown to reduce anxiety, one of the main reasons for sleep difficulty. So drink up and soak it in, the calming effects of tea are scientifically supported!

Journal Writing

We've all heard that we need an outlet. Well, writing is one of them. By keeping a journal, you can significantly reduce your ability to focus on negativity. And when you're not worry about negativity, you're less likely to toss and turn. Just be careful, studies indicate that journaling about emotions alone may have a negative effect. It's best to write out in your journals both the emotions that bother you and how you think about them. By pairing cognitive with emotional, we are better prepared for navigating the dark waters of our inner feelings.

Turn the Alarm Clock

When you can't fall asleep, you start to worry more. You remind yourself that you need sleep, and that the next day is going to be even rougher as a result. Then, you start staring at the alarm clock. Unfortunately, this only makes falling asleep even harder. Not to mention, artificial light from electronic gadgets messes with our circadian rhythms. So don't let out artificial lights in the dark—and don't obsess over what time it is!

Technology to the Rescue

We use our smartphones for everything nowadays. So why not use them for tracking our sleep? New apps allow our smartphones to track our sleep patterns and quality while we doze off. Over time, this permits us to learn what does and doesn't work. So get into it!

Cherry Juice

Studies show that consuming tart cherry juice concentrate is good for ushering in sleep. It is believed that the phytochemicals in tart cherry juice help to increase exogenous melatonin levels in the body. Because melatonin is naturally produced to fall asleep, this helps us get the shut-eye we need. So drink up!

Time your Meals and Drinks

Some people report going into a "food coma" following large meals. This may help in certain cases, but it is also important to remember not to eat so much as to get indigestion. Furthermore, make sure you are well-hydrated prior to going to sleep so that you don't wake up thirsty. It's important not to take these measures too far, as too much food or liquid may lead to insomnia. Your best bet is to try what's worked for you in the past, as you know your body best. Eating dairy foods and carbohydrates may be the quickest way to ease into sleep.

Exercise

Exercise is always a big one, but only if done at the right time. Exercise stimulates the body to secrete the stress hormone cortisol, which triggers the brain's alerting mechanism. Do your last bout of exercise at least three hours prior to bedtime. By this point, the effect of your workout will have induced fatigue and you'll be happy to drift off to sleep.

Lavender

Some studies indicate that lavender-scented candles or essential oils are indispensable when it comes to beating insomnia. This choice beats hypnotic agents which have potentially serious adverse effects on the brain and body. So go lavender, and go natural!

Beat "Blue light"

Most electronic devices emit "blue light," which is a main reason for sleep disturbances. Although light of any kind can suppress the secretion of the all-important melatonin, blue light is the most powerful. Harvard researchers found that exposure to 6.5 hours of blue light suppressed melatonin for about twice as long as green light exposure. Exposure also offset circadian rhythms by twice as much (3 hrs. compared to 1.5 hrs). If dimming the lights and repositioning electronic devices doesn't work, you might want to try specially designed glasses for blocking blue light.

Keep the Pet at Bay

Sure, you might enjoy snuggling with your little bundle of fur, but research shows that ultimately you'll pay the price. When snuggling with a pet during the night, that pet moves as you move. Paired with another person in your bed and you've got a recipe for sleep disturbance. Moving your pet from the bed is not betrayal. Your pet won't care and you'll end up enjoying higher quality sleep. More peace and more comfort. Isn't that what you want?

Wear Socks

Warm feet -- a sign of healthy blood flow – are important for quality sleep. By warming up cold feet, through cozy socks, you will also warm up your whole body. Don't let heat escape through your extremities! Keep your thermoregulation under control and ensure your blood flow is doing well.

Zinc-Magnesium

If you want to go the supplement route, taking ZMA is believed to have many health benefits. It works for both workout recovery and sleep quality control. If you aren't up to taking supplements, eating leafy greens like spinach, and nuts such as almonds or magnesium, and meat/shellfish are the easiest ways to get both minerals. If you do choose supplements over foods, however, be sure to aim for aspartate.

White-out Noise

No matter where you live, there is going to be *some* noise when you go to sleep. If you can't possibly eliminate the noise pollution, your next best bet is to use white-noise machines. These devices are actually sound-producing devices. By simply pressing a button, a white-noise machine issues a soft, whooshing noise that drowns out the majority of sudden and unpredictable noises that disturb our sleep. The advanced models can produce the sounds of rain, wind, waves or other natural ambient noises. The volume of these machines is constant and soft so it doesn't wake you up. White-out machines usually run from $50 to $150.

Caffeine Control

Make sure you keep drinking caffeine to the mornings. Even if you are a regular drinker, consuming too much soda, coffee, or other caffeine-loaded substances may keep you up. Unless you're trying to pull an all-nighter, consuming caffeine close to bedtime is a no-no.

Sleep Hygiene

Maintaining good sleep habits is important. Studies show that poor sleepers exhibit an increased level of cognitive activity in the bed, even after controlling for depression and anxiety problems. Poor sleepers have excessive noise in the bedroom, intolerable nighttime temperatures, and activities that demanded high concentration prior to bedtime. So basically, if you want to practice good "sleep hygiene," *don't* do those things!

Sun and Air

Circadian rhythms are the rhythms that dictate our minds and bodies. In a world without artificial lighting, before all this technology, our ancestors woke with the sun and fell asleep to the rising moon. Exposure to daylight will regulate the internal clock. By getting some sunlight and fresh air, we keep daytime fatigue at bay, thus ensuring the onset of sleepiness around nightfall.

Don't Force It

Too many times, people tell themselves they have to go to sleep and then they try to *will* themselves into it. Unfortunately, this usually occurs after a day's worth of activities that has prepared us *not* to be able to fall asleep when we want to. Instead of struggling to fall asleep, getting frustrated, and struggling further—give yourself 20 minutes. If you're not asleep after 20 minutes, get out of bed, go to another room, and do something calming like reading a book or listening to music. Don't think about sleeping; let it come naturally.

No Alcohol or Nicotine

If you find that you need your 'fix,' save if for earlier in the day. Or better yet, work on quitting altogether. Nicotine is a stimulant, and alcohol acts as one as well, even if it may help to bring on sleep initially. Limit alcohol consumption to two to three drinks per day, or at the very least, don't drink within three hours of bedtime.

Dinner by Candlelight

Candlelit dinners are more than romantic meals; they actually soothe the body, especially after workouts. Ditching artificial lighting and replacing them with candles can do wonders—not to mention it changes up the ambience. Fire emits very little blue light, especially little tiny flames. This characteristic of candlelight offers a unique physiological advantage. Your body rests naturally.

Get More Thiamine

Don't know what thiamine is? Basically, it's found in meat, especially pork, and is a major player in quality sleep. If you don't get enough, your sleep may suffer. If you love bacon, you're in luck. Sunflower seeds are also high in thiamine.

Massage or Foam Roll

It would be nice if we all had personal massage therapists, but hey, ain't life a bitch? If your partner is not hitting the right spots, have him or her focus on the shoulders, the lower back, and the legs. You can also foam roll yourself which will release a lot of physical and mental tension to make sleep more satisfying. Focus on legs and upper back for ten minutes before going to bed. You'll feel loose and limber!

Taurine

Here's another one you might not know. If you've had energy drinks before, you might have noticed this listed on the ingredients label. Ironically, Taurine actually has sedative effects. Taurine is a non-essential amino acid, but is still <u>very important</u> when pertaining to sleep. Taurine plays a role in activation of GABA, a prevalent neurotransmitter linked to sleepiness.

When it comes to getting more Taurine in your diet, you might just have to mix things up. If you've never eaten animal hearts before, now's the time to try. The thought may disgust you, but just think about all the other animals' parts you might have eaten—without really even knowing it. Besides, animal hearts are healthy, tasty, and tender. Turkey and grass-feed beef hearts can be found at many Whole Foods markets.

Harness Stress

This one's a no-brainer, but not enough people actually know how to do it. Instead of focusing on completely eliminating stress, try to <u>harness the stress you have</u>. When you experience periods of acute stress, use them to your advantage. Work harder, think smarter, become more creative, and channel your emotions and thoughts positively. Studies show that acute stress has many benefits through what is called "hormesis," so long as it doesn't reach chronic, unmanageable levels.

So don't stress your stress! Harness it!

Check Your Medications

There's a laundry list of medications that may affect your ability to sleep soundly. Beta-blockers for hypertension can cause insomnia, as can Selective Serotonin Reuptake Inhibitors (SSRIs) for depression, such as Zoloft and Prozac. If you are taking any other medicine, make your list and check with your doctor. Who knows what those pills and gelatins may be doing to your biochemistry!

The Sleep Snack

Experts say that the perfect nighttime snack should have both carbohydrates and either calcium or a protein containing tryptophan. Tryptophan is an amino acid that is found in turkey, which makes us sleepy. It makes us sleepy because it boosts levels of the neurotransmitter serotonin in our brain. Serotonin makes us feel calm, so if you're trying to fall asleep and want something to eat, have a light snack an hour before bedtime to give the tryptophan time to settle in.

Experts recommend:

§ Whole grain cereal and fat-free milk, or

§ Fruit and low-fat yogurt

§ Whole grain toast with a slice of low-fat cheese or turkey

§ Banana with a small amount of peanut butter

Pillow Position

Ever toss and turn, trying desperately to find that perfect position for your head and body? If you're struggling with this, remember one thing: the perfect prop for your head will keep your spine and neck aligned in a straight line. This will prevent tension or cramps that keep you from falling asleep. If your neck is flexed back or raised, find a pillow that lets you sleep in a better position. If you're a stomach sleeper, use either no pillow or a very flat one to keep everything straight.

Pajamas Please

Some people like to sleep naked or very scantly clothed. However, experts recommend pajamas. Research shows that warm skin helps to slows down your blood's circulation, cools your internal temp., and generally contributes to deeper more rejuvenating sleep. Because our bodies go through several cool-warm cycles as the night progresses, sheets, covers, and clothes that keep you comfortable are the way to go.

Deep Breathing

Sort of like meditation, this helps reduce your heart rate and blood pressure, releases feel-good endorphins, and relaxes your body, better preparing you for sleep. To practice deep breathing, simply: inhale for 5 seconds, then pause for 3, then exhale for 5. Repeat 10 times at first, then work your way to 15. To see if you're doing it right, use a bottle of children's bubbles and blow through the wand. The same breath used in blowing successful bubbles should be used in deep breathing. Make sure you breathe using your belly.

Know Your Cycle

No, I'm not talking about menstrual cycle. By knowing your sleeping cycle, you will dramatically improve your chances of healthy sleep. Do you ever find you get really sleepy at a certain time? Does your spell of sleepiness come and then you're wide awake? If this sounds like you, it's good to plan ahead. Know when this happens, and get ready for sleep before it fully settles in. Otherwise, you might *just* be up all night.

Well there you have it. If none of these tips help you to drift off to dreamland, nothing will! By applying these strategies, remember to also make important lifestyle changes. Eat healthier foods, exercise daily, and harness your stress. It is important that you take every opportunity to do daytime activities... during the daytime. Unless you can function by being nocturnal, it's probably best to make nighttime a time for unwinding.

Okay, so let's say you've figured it out. You're well-rested, feeling healthy, and looking forward to sleep because you know it's good. But this doesn't stop you from having other questions. Such as... well, what the heck is this whole *dreaming* thing about any way? Forget just sleeping, why do we dream? Are our strange and sometimes completely mundane visions something important or are they just the ramblings of an unconscious world?

Dream Theory: Understanding Why We Dream

Truth be told, dreaming continues to be one of behavioral sciences' greatest unanswered questions. Ancient civilizations believed dreams were portals through which the gods gave divine wisdom. Egyptians used them to make future predictions. In more recent times, the role of dreams as the expression of the unconscious desire has been popularized by psychologist Sigmund Freud. To this day, shamans use dreams to treat illnesses, believing the unconscious mind recognizes illnesses well before the conscious mind.

Although many theories have been conjured, there is still no single unifying one. Over the last century or so, there have been four major dream theories.

Let's take a look:

The No Meaning Theory

As the name suggests, this theory posits that dreams have no deeper meaning. Basically, it is all just the random firing of impulses as our brain goes about its nightly ritual. This is supported by scanning of sleeping people's brains during REM sleep. This challenges Freud's idea of dreams as symbolically meaningful. The main points of this are:

- Dreaming is a physiological anomaly not a psychological function

- Images and sounds in dreams are merely manifestation of brain's signals

- Ultimately random and meaningless

Of course, other theories challenge this by showing that there is a purpose and function to dreaming. For many, the elaborate structure of dream worlds and sequences suggests a deeper meaning.

The Organization Theory

This theory suggests that dreaming serves the critical function of de-cluttering the brain. Because our brains are slammed with conscious and unconscious stimuli all throughout the day, dreaming helps to make sense of the mess. The main points are:

- Dreaming is a way to keep new information and release irrelevant information

- Dreaming organizes the brain and optimizes learning

- Dreaming replays the events of the day

Those who argue against this theory assert that dreaming is not filing because our brains are not computers. They also point out that most of our dreams do not relate to our daily lives. While there may be some 'day residue,' for the most part, dreams are strange and fantastical.

The Problem-Solving Theory

This theory contends that dreams are great for finding solutions to problems that go untreated during the day. Basically:

- Dreaming registers subtleties that are consciously missed

- Dreaming rewires our brain to find new solutions

- Dreaming creates wisdom

Many who contest this theory believe that dreaming is not nearly so useful. Firstly, many medications that suppress REM sleep do not in fact cause memory problems. Most importantly, we usually don't remember our dreams… many of us forget the dreams as soon as we open our eyes… So then what *exactly* are we learning? And how can we solve a problem if we don't remember the solution? Those who argue against this point state that we may be gaining unconscious insights; that the answers to our solutions arrive from dreaming without us knowing where they came from. Sort of like an "Ah-hah!" moment.

The Coping Theory

Some experts believe that dreaming may be a form of traumatic coping, or psychotherapy. Based on our emotions, we all have dreams to cope with certain situations, circumstances, feelings, or thoughts. You may dream of deaths, of accidents, of failures and fears—many times we dream of bad things that happened or are likely to happen. It is through this dreaming, experts say, that we learn to cope with those problems should they come again. The main points are:

- Dreaming confronts difficult emotions in a new way

- Dreaming puts our emotions in pictures and visions

·   Dreaming allows us to accept truths our waking, defensive brains might deny

Of course, this theory doesn't really explain why we dream of fantastical or extremely mundane things. But it does suggest that nightmares can be a type of preparation or rehearsal for trauma.

So then…

Now that we have an idea of what dreaming might actually mean, the purpose it might serve, we have another task ahead. That is, it's time to make sense of our dreams. It's time to plunge deep into the dreamscape.

Delving Deep: Interpreting Your Dreamscape

You've probably woken up some mornings, shaking your head, wondering what the *heck* you just dreamt... and why. Well, the answer is never easy, but if you put in a little work, you can definitely make sense of your strangest dreams. Heck, you can even begin to apply their messages to the waking world.

Remember, the dreams are your subconscious mind making stuff happen. There is usually an absence of logic. You aren't using your higher thinking—you are instead going along for a topsy-turvy ride. Emotions and thoughts; fears and securities; doubts and certainties; all of these things factor into our dreams.

Dreams can be thought of as the influx of everything we've taught our brains throughout our lives. We may notice various concepts that recur in many of our visions. If you see repetitive imagery, or experience similar feelings, from dream to dream—figure out what it means!

If you're constantly falling or slipping or losing control in your dreams, your mind might be telling you that you need to get your life on track. If you, however, seem to be commanding your dreams, or exercising great power, then maybe your mind is telling you've that you've got everything on lock-down.

Remember, these are *your* dreams. Any so-called 'dream rules' may not apply, so it is up to you to learn what your dreams might mean. When it comes to interpreting dream symbols, think deep and hard. Recall your past, consider recent events—even events that occurred literally right before you feel asleep. It is even possible that external stimuli may figure into your dreams. A roaming cat in your bedroom may be a feline beast in your dreams; a rain shower outside your window may become a flood in your dream world.

Consider the possibilities, be open-minded, and use your dreams for good. If you think you can apply the lessons learned, do so. However, if you still don't know what *the heck* your dreams are about, don't worry. For a definitive guide to dream symbols, try Cloud Nine.

It might just change your life.

But even if it doesn't, it will certainly offer some insight into the crazy world of the human dreamscape. And speaking of dreamscape, if you're *really* interested in remembering and analyzing your dreams, it's time to step up your game.

Create a dream diary that allows you to:

1. Identify Symbols – Notice how many times certain symbols appear and document them. Then analyze their underlying meaning. Over time, tally up how often certain symbols appear in your journal. If you want to really understand your dreams, also document minor and major events during the days that may have impacted your dreams.

2. Improve Recall – One way to remember dreams is to set your alarm clock to wake you following each REM cycle: after the first three hours, then every 90 minutes. Because this disrupts your sleep, don't do it too often. You'll be astonished how often you remember your dreams.

3. Deepen Meaning – Writing and talking about dreams will prime your mind. If you consciously tell it to remember more dreams, it will. Amazingly. This will also open up new communication channels with your subconscious, making dream analysis more feasible and meaningful—pretty cool, huh?

Okay, so even if you know how to keep a proper dream diary, it might help to have a little more background about common symbols. If you're wondering what dreams mean, take a deeper look. Go into the world of dreaming and make it happen. Better yet, gain a grasp on the most important and prevalent dream symbols known to man….

The Top 20 Dream Symbols

There are a lot of weird images that pop up in our dreams. Sometimes they are so 'out there,' we may wonder if they have any real meaning at all. Other times, we can quickly uncover the significance. Here is a list of some of the most common dream symbols and what they may mean to you:

1. **Babies** may symbolize a desire to reproduce. The human infant may also represent a need to start anew, or a certain level of vulnerability.

2. **Animals** represent a natural connection. They might also hint at a definite repression or suppression of 'animalistic' desires. Perhaps, you want to live on the wild side?

3. **Clothes** reflect how we want to be perceived. Shoddy clothes in our dreams may be a figurative way of saying we feel worn out or misrepresented. Nice clothes may indicate a certain confidence or success.

4. **Exams** can represent self-reflection or perhaps, external pressures from those around us. Maybe we feel like we're being unfairly assessed?

5. **Death** is a common one. It can mean the end or beginning of a new phase or lifestyle. It may be the subconscious way of dealing with a recent passing. Or it may simply represent a general consideration of

human mortality.

6. **Falling** represents the anxiety of letting go, of feeling helpless or no longer supported. It may hint at our perceived inability to do what we want the way we want it.

7. **Food** is said to be a representation of knowledge. We 'consume' information to grow and prosper.

8. **Demons** are dark, deceptive entities that often signify a deeper insecurity or issue. Our mind may be telling us that it's time to sort through the darkness in our lives.

9. **Hair** is, according to Freud, related to sexuality. Losing hair in a dream may be a loss of libido or the actual fear of losing hair. Lots of hair may represent sexual potency.

10. **Houses** contain other dream symbols, but the building itself is typically considered as a representation of the inner psyche. Each room or floor may hint at your various emotions, memories and interpretations.

11. **Killing** may represent the desire to exterminate a part of your personality or way of life. It may also represent a hostility or ill-will toward a person or people.

12. **Marriage** can be the 'union' of the male and/or female faculties, or a desire to actually get married.

13. **Money** may symbolize self-worth and other forms of self-appraisal. Money transactions in dreams sometimes signify the need to exchange a part of oneself for something else.

14.**Mountains** are typically obstacles to be conquered. Reach the pinnacle represents conquering demons, achieving goals, and/or starting anew. Failing in the face of the mountain may mean that you are struggling with a major obstacle in your life.

15.**Nudity** is a common one. Plenty of people have had dreams of being nude in front of others. Typically, this means that you are exposing your true self or have become vulnerable. You may also simply have unmet sexual desires.

16.**Roads** are not only literal paths, but also figurative paths. They may represent the right path or the wrong path, or the uncertain path, depending upon how they appear and what happens along them.

17.**Sex** dreams may represent a need for 'getting some'. Many times, however, sexual imagery means that we are conceiving of new possibilities, new avenues, and new attitudes.

18.**Teeth** show up a lot. If your teeth rot or fall out, you're probably fearing that you may be getting cavities, are losing your 'bite,' or you're simply afraid of getting older.

19.**Feeling Trapped** is a prevalent theme, reflecting your real life inability to move on or rid yourself of something unwanted.

20.**Water** has many shapes, sizes, and functions in dreams, just like in real life. In the subconscious mind, calm pools of water mean harmony, while an uneasy ocean can mean that you're internally unstable.

Now that you have a grasp of what your dreams might mean, you can certainly move on. Rest assured, you will probably never look at dreams quite the same way again. Instead, you'll move on with confidence and faith, knowing that things can and do get better, if just briefly, where sleep is concerned. You'll have a better understanding of yourself, of what you need to change, and how you can change it.

But what about that other part of sleeping that isn't *quite* sleeping?

What about naps?

The Incredible Power of the Power Nap: Your Guide to a 'Quickie'

For the longest time, people considered napping to be a bad habit—an excuse for the sleep-deprived to shoo away their daily demands and depart briefly to the world of shuteye. Fortunately, the stigma is now fading, as the science grows clearer. Truth be told, so-called 'power naps' not only alleviate sleep deficits, but are also great ways to boost our cerebral functioning, including gains in creative problem solving, verbal memory, perceptual learning, object learning, and statistical learning (that's a lot of learning).

Power naps improve our skills when it comes to math, logical reasoning, reaction, and symbolic recognition. Not to mention, naps get rid of negative moods associated with fatigue and sleepiness. Moreover, napping has scientifically supported benefits for the heart, our blood pressure, our stress levels, and even weight control.

In the world of napping, there are multiple types. There are naps of 10-20 minute duration, the typical power nap. They usually occur between 1 and 4 p.m. and give us that burst of wakefulness we need for functioning till bedtime. There are also micro-naps that last a scant 5 or 6 minutes and can provide short jolts of energy and improved ability to recall facts and knowledge. Then there are longer naps that last an hour or 90 minutes, and can improve our cognitive skills in processing memories. Naps are typically one of four types:

- **Scheduled napping**: Also known as planned napping, these rest periods involve taking a nap prior to getting sleepy. It's a good thing to do in preparation for a late night.

- **Emergency napping**: This is the kind of must-have nap when we're simply too tired to do what we have to do. In certain circumstances, emergency napping is advisable to actually continuing what we're doing. Such as in the case of operating machinery or performing important and difficult cognitive tasks.

- **Habitual napping**: When we take a nap the same time every day.

- **Appetitive napping**: When we nap because we, well, simply like it.

Let's quickly review how these naps are effective.

All naps have their benefits, especially planned naps. Planned naps actually improve alertness and performance for those who have to be on high-alert for intense situations. This includes emergency department physicians and nurses, as well as first-year medical students. Naps can rejuvenate our attention, improve the quality of our work, and reduce our likelihood for mistakes. They also improve our ability to learn.

In fact, naps are so powerful, that some studies have shown they can improve verbal memory, motor skills, and perceptual learning better than caffeine. Moreover, caffeine is linked to reduction in motor sequence learning and declarative verbal memory. Power naps are not.

Naps can have also been associated with greater rates of stress reduction. This is very important and explains why napping also impacts blood pressure for the better. Naps accelerate cardiovascular recovery after bouts of stress. A simple 45 minute nap <u>measurably lowers blood pressure.</u> And not to mention, <u>sheds weight</u>—another contributor to high blood pressure.

Naps also have long-term benefits. One longitudinal study followed almost 24,000 people over a 6-year period. None of them had any health issues related to heart disease, stroke, or cancer, and by the study's conclusion, those napping three times a week showed a 37% lower chance of dying from a heart-related disease.

In conclusion, napping is awesome. It is great for the mind and body, great for preventing diseases and illnesses, great for simply feeling good, and great for those who aren't living as healthily and as happily as they wish. Put simply, you *should* nap, if only from time to time. Who knows, maybe it will counteract some of your *other*, less-than-stellar habits…

And speaking of habits, when it comes to sleeping—in general—it comes down to habit. If you're struggling with falling asleep, if your lifestyle is getting the better of you, if things simply aren't lining up the way you want them to, there is always change. You can change your sleeping habits, and patterns; you can change the way you perceive sleeping; you can change your waking schedule, and everything in between the time you wake up and the time you put your weary head on that pillow. Maybe it's as simple as looking at your dreams…

Bottom line is: we control our own destinies. We decide what we want to do with the time we have, for the most part. If you're not sleeping well and it's affecting your life, you have the power to change it. You can consult with a doctor or expert, you can do the research, you can read informative books such as this one, and you can make the conscious choice to move forward. The move is yours, and the power is in your hands.

So take that power, take that electric surge, and hit the switch.

Turn it to "Off." It's beddy-bye time.

***

A Special Note:

Thank you for reading "*Deep Sleep: 32 Proven Tips for Deeper, Longer, More Rejuvenating Sleep.*" If you enjoyed reading this book and would like to be included on an email list for when similar content is available, feel free:

SUBSCRIBE

As always, thank you for reading.

And may you continue to live healthily and happily.

Sincerely,

C.K. Murray

Other works by C.K. Murray:

1. *Mindfulness Explained: The Mindful Solution to Stress, Depression, and Chronic Unhappiness*

2. *Emotional Intelligence Explained: How to Master Emotional Intelligence and Unlock Your True Ability*

34. BEAT The Hangover: Your Ultimate Guide to Drinking, Partying and Waking up Hangover Free

Made in the USA
San Bernardino, CA
03 February 2019